CONTENTS

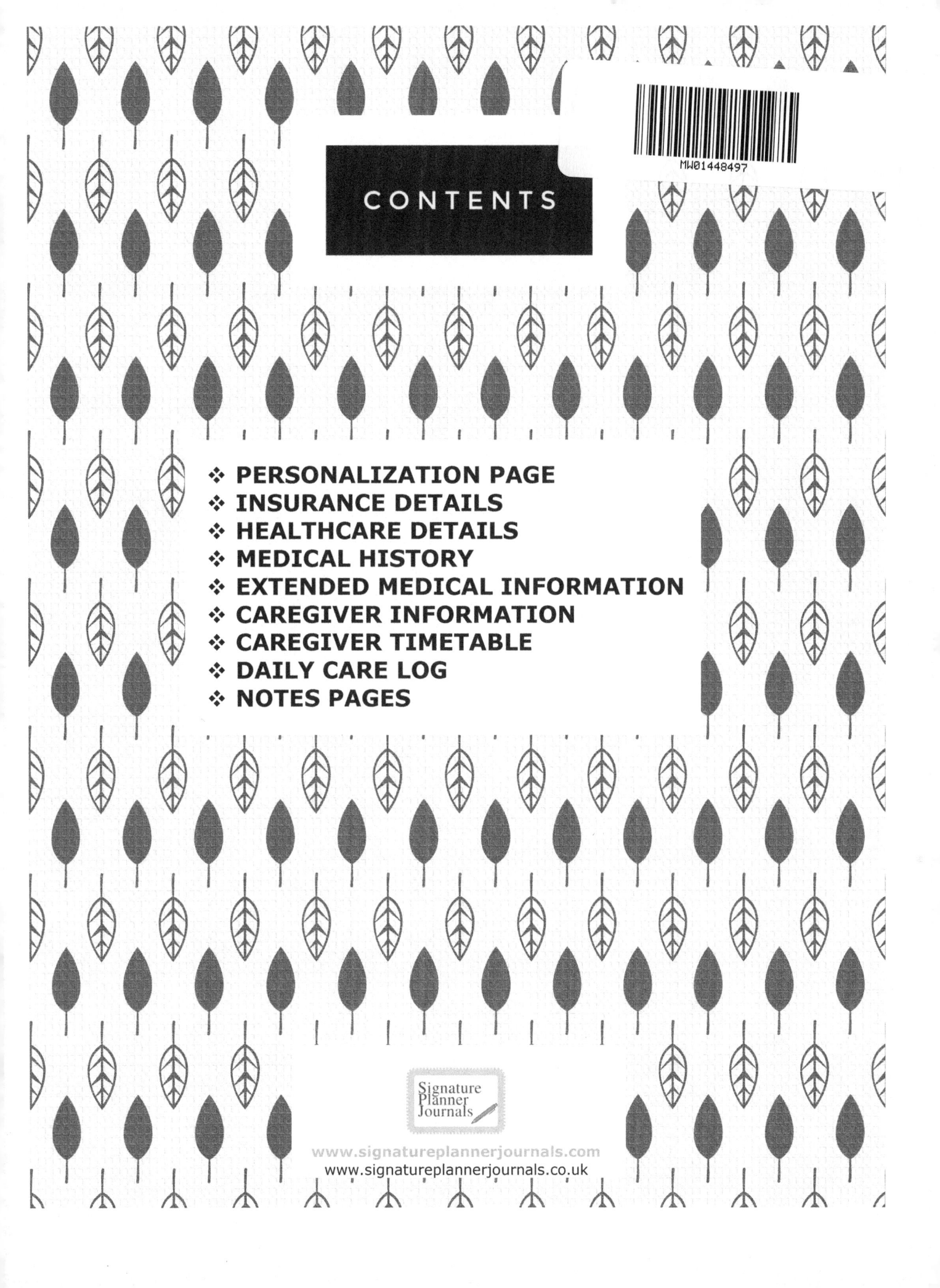

- **PERSONALIZATION PAGE**
- **INSURANCE DETAILS**
- **HEALTHCARE DETAILS**
- **MEDICAL HISTORY**
- **EXTENDED MEDICAL INFORMATION**
- **CAREGIVER INFORMATION**
- **CAREGIVER TIMETABLE**
- **DAILY CARE LOG**
- **NOTES PAGES**

Signature Planner Journals

www.signatureplannerjournals.com
www.signatureplannerjournals.co.uk

NAME			AGE	
CONTACT No.				
ADDRESS				
ALLERGIES				
PHYSICIAN				
Contact Number				
Address				

EMERGENCY CONTACTS	
Contact Number	
Emergency Contact	Name
Contact Number	
Emergency Contact	Name
Contact Number	

REGULAR MEDICATION

NAME OF MEDICATION		Date Started	Dated Ended	DOSE
Purpose	**Shape**	**Color**	**Special Instructions**	

NAME OF MEDICATION		Date Started	Dated Ended	DOSE
Purpose	**Shape**	**Color**	**Special Instructions**	

NAME OF MEDICATION		Date Started	Dated Ended	DOSE
Purpose	**Shape**	**Color**	**Special Instructions**	

NOTES

INSURANCE DETAILS

COMPANY	
POLICY START DATE	POLICY END DATE
COVER DETAILS	
ADDRESS	
CONTACT NO.	
EMAIL	
WEBSITE	

COMPANY	
POLICY START DATE	POLICY END DATE
COVER DETAILS	
ADDRESS	
CONTACT NO.	
EMAIL	
WEBSITE	

COMPANY	
POLICY START DATE	POLICY END DATE
COVER DETAILS	
ADDRESS	
CONTACT NO.	
EMAIL	
WEBSITE	

COMPANY	
POLICY START DATE	POLICY END DATE
COVER DETAILS	
ADDRESS	
CONTACT NO.	
EMAIL	
WEBSITE	

HEALTH CARE DETAILS

PEDIATRICIAN DETAILS
NAME:
ADDRESS:

PHONE NUMBER:

DENTIST
NAME:
ADDRESS:

PHONE NUMBER:

SPECIALIST
NAME:
DETAILS:
ADDRESS:

PHONE NUMBER:

SPECIALIST
NAME:
DETAILS:
ADDRESS:

PHONE NUMBER:

SPECIALIST
NAME:
DETAILS:
ADDRESS:

PHONE NUMBER:

SPECIALIST
NAME:
DETAILS:
ADDRESS:

PHONE NUMBER:

SPECIALIST
NAME:
DETAILS:
ADDRESS:

PHONE NUMBER:

MEDICAL HISTORY

	YES	NO	NOTES
High Blood Pressure			
Stroke			
High Cholesterol			
Diabetes			
Glaucoma			
Epilepsy			
Asthma			
Obesity			
Allergies			
Cancer (type)			
Hearing Loss			
Alcohol Misuse			
Drug Misuse			
Kidney Problems			
Incontinent			
Ambulant			
	YES	NO	NOTES

EXTENDED MEDICAL INFORMATION

CAREGIVER INFORMATION

NAME	
ORGANISATION	
RELATIONSHIP	
CONTACT No.	
EMAIL	
ADDRESS	

TYPE OF ASSISTANCE	Personal Care		Cleaning		Meal Prep.	
	Medication		Shopping		Transportation	
	Appointments		Paying Bills		Other	
FREQUENCY OF VISITS	Daily		Weekly		Fortnightly		Monthly	

NOTES

NAME	
ORGANISATION	
RELATIONSHIP	
CONTACT No.	
EMAIL	
ADDRESS	

TYPE OF ASSISTANCE	Personal Care		Cleaning		Meal Prep.	
	Medication		Shopping		Transportation	
	Appointments		Paying Bills		Other	
FREQUENCY OF VISITS	Daily		Weekly		Fortnightly		Monthly	

NOTES

CAREGIVER INFORMATION

NAME	
ORGANISATION	
RELATIONSHIP	
CONTACT No.	
EMAIL	
ADDRESS	

TYPE OF ASSISTANCE	Personal Care		Cleaning		Meal Prep.	
	Medication		Shopping		Transportation	
	Appointments		Paying Bills		Other	
FREQUENCY OF VISITS	**Daily**		**Weekly**		**Fortnightly**	**Monthly**

NOTES	

NAME	
ORGANISATION	
RELATIONSHIP	
CONTACT No.	
EMAIL	
ADDRESS	

TYPE OF ASSISTANCE	Personal Care		Cleaning		Meal Prep.	
	Medication		Shopping		Transportation	
	Appointments		Paying Bills		Other	
FREQUENCY OF VISITS	**Daily**		**Weekly**		**Fortnightly**	**Monthly**

NOTES	

CAREGIVER INFORMATION

NAME	
ORGANISATION	
RELATIONSHIP	
CONTACT No.	
EMAIL	
ADDRESS	

TYPE OF ASSISTANCE	Personal Care		Cleaning		Meal Prep.	
	Medication		Shopping		Transportation	
	Appointments		Paying Bills		Other	
FREQUENCY OF VISITS	Daily		Weekly		Fortnightly		Monthly	

NOTES

NAME	
ORGANISATION	
RELATIONSHIP	
CONTACT No.	
EMAIL	
ADDRESS	

TYPE OF ASSISTANCE	Personal Care		Cleaning		Meal Prep.	
	Medication		Shopping		Transportation	
	Appointments		Paying Bills		Other	
FREQUENCY OF VISITS	Daily		Weekly		Fortnightly		Monthly	

NOTES

CAREGIVER INFORMATION

NAME	
ORGANISATION	
RELATIONSHIP	
CONTACT No.	
EMAIL	
ADDRESS	

TYPE OF ASSISTANCE	Personal Care		Cleaning		Meal Prep.	
	Medication		Shopping		Transportation	
	Appointments		Paying Bills		Other	
FREQUENCY OF VISITS	**Daily**		**Weekly**		**Fortnightly**		**Monthly**	

NOTES

NAME	
ORGANISATION	
RELATIONSHIP	
CONTACT No.	
EMAIL	
ADDRESS	

TYPE OF ASSISTANCE	Personal Care		Cleaning		Meal Prep.	
	Medication		Shopping		Transportation	
	Appointments		Paying Bills		Other	
FREQUENCY OF VISITS	**Daily**		**Weekly**		**Fortnightly**		**Monthly**	

NOTES

CAREGIVER INFORMATION

NAME	
ORGANISATION	
RELATIONSHIP	
CONTACT No.	
EMAIL	
ADDRESS	

TYPE OF ASSISTANCE	Personal Care		Cleaning		Meal Prep.	
	Medication		Shopping		Transportation	
	Appointments		Paying Bills		Other	
FREQUENCY OF VISITS	Daily		Weekly		Fortnightly		Monthly	

NOTES

NAME	
ORGANISATION	
RELATIONSHIP	
CONTACT No.	
EMAIL	
ADDRESS	

TYPE OF ASSISTANCE	Personal Care		Cleaning		Meal Prep.	
	Medication		Shopping		Transportation	
	Appointments		Paying Bills		Other	
FREQUENCY OF VISITS	Daily		Weekly		Fortnightly		Monthly	

NOTES

CAREGIVER INFORMATION

NAME	
ORGANISATION	
RELATIONSHIP	
CONTACT No.	
EMAIL	
ADDRESS	

TYPE OF ASSISTANCE	Personal Care		Cleaning		Meal Prep.	
	Medication		Shopping		Transportation	
	Appointments		Paying Bills		Other	
FREQUENCY OF VISITS	**Daily**		**Weekly**		**Fortnightly**	**Monthly**

NOTES

NAME	
ORGANISATION	
RELATIONSHIP	
CONTACT No.	
EMAIL	
ADDRESS	

TYPE OF ASSISTANCE	Personal Care		Cleaning		Meal Prep.	
	Medication		Shopping		Transportation	
	Appointments		Paying Bills		Other	
FREQUENCY OF VISITS	**Daily**		**Weekly**		**Fortnightly**	**Monthly**

NOTES

CAREGIVER TIMETABLE

CAREGIVER NAME							
DATE							
🕐	MON	TUES	WED	THRS	FRI	SAT	SUN
START							
FINISH							
TOTAL Hrs							

CAREGIVER NAME							
DATE							
🕐	MON	TUES	WED	THRS	FRI	SAT	SUN
START							
FINISH							
TOTAL Hrs							

CAREGIVER NAME							
DATE							
🕐	MON	TUES	WED	THRS	FRI	SAT	SUN
START							
FINISH							
TOTAL Hrs							

CAREGIVER NAME							
DATE							
🕐	MON	TUES	WED	THRS	FRI	SAT	SUN
START							
FINISH							
TOTAL Hrs							

_____

_____

_____

_____

CAREGIVER TIMETABLE

CAREGIVER NAME							
DATE							
🕐	MON	TUES	WED	THRS	FRI	SAT	SUN
START							
FINISH							
TOTAL Hrs							

CAREGIVER NAME							
DATE							
🕐	MON	TUES	WED	THRS	FRI	SAT	SUN
START							
FINISH							
TOTAL Hrs							

CAREGIVER NAME							
DATE							
🕐	MON	TUES	WED	THRS	FRI	SAT	SUN
START							
FINISH							
TOTAL Hrs							

CAREGIVER NAME							
DATE							
🕐	MON	TUES	WED	THRS	FRI	SAT	SUN
START							
FINISH							
TOTAL Hrs							

_____

_____

_____

CAREGIVER TIMETABLE

CAREGIVER NAME							
DATE							
🕒	MON	TUES	WED	THRS	FRI	SAT	SUN
START							
FINISH							
TOTAL Hrs							

CAREGIVER NAME							
DATE							
🕒	MON	TUES	WED	THRS	FRI	SAT	SUN
START							
FINISH							
TOTAL Hrs							

CAREGIVER NAME							
DATE							
🕒	MON	TUES	WED	THRS	FRI	SAT	SUN
START							
FINISH							
TOTAL Hrs							

CAREGIVER NAME							
DATE							
🕒	MON	TUES	WED	THRS	FRI	SAT	SUN
START							
FINISH							
TOTAL Hrs							

_____

_____

_____

CAREGIVER TIMETABLE

CAREGIVER NAME							
DATE							
🕐	MON	TUES	WED	THRS	FRI	SAT	SUN
START							
FINISH							
TOTAL Hrs							

CAREGIVER NAME							
DATE							
🕐	MON	TUES	WED	THRS	FRI	SAT	SUN
START							
FINISH							
TOTAL Hrs							

CAREGIVER NAME							
DATE							
🕐	MON	TUES	WED	THRS	FRI	SAT	SUN
START							
FINISH							
TOTAL Hrs							

CAREGIVER NAME							
DATE							
🕐	MON	TUES	WED	THRS	FRI	SAT	SUN
START							
FINISH							
TOTAL Hrs							

_____

_____

_____

CAREGIVER TIMETABLE

CAREGIVER NAME

DATE 🕐	MON	TUES	WED	THRS	FRI	SAT	SUN
START							
FINISH							
TOTAL Hrs							

CAREGIVER NAME

DATE 🕐	MON	TUES	WED	THRS	FRI	SAT	SUN
START							
FINISH							
TOTAL Hrs							

CAREGIVER NAME

DATE 🕐	MON	TUES	WED	THRS	FRI	SAT	SUN
START							
FINISH							
TOTAL Hrs							

CAREGIVER NAME

DATE 🕐	MON	TUES	WED	THRS	FRI	SAT	SUN
START							
FINISH							
TOTAL Hrs							

_____
_____
_____

CAREGIVER TIMETABLE

CAREGIVER NAME							
DATE							
🕐	MON	TUES	WED	THRS	FRI	SAT	SUN
START							
FINISH							
TOTAL Hrs							

CAREGIVER NAME							
DATE							
🕐	MON	TUES	WED	THRS	FRI	SAT	SUN
START							
FINISH							
TOTAL Hrs							

CAREGIVER NAME							
DATE							
🕐	MON	TUES	WED	THRS	FRI	SAT	SUN
START							
FINISH							
TOTAL Hrs							

CAREGIVER NAME							
DATE							
🕐	MON	TUES	WED	THRS	FRI	SAT	SUN
START							
FINISH							
TOTAL Hrs							

_____

_____

_____

CAREGIVER TIMETABLE

CAREGIVER NAME							
DATE							
🕒	MON	TUES	WED	THRS	FRI	SAT	SUN
START							
FINISH							
TOTAL Hrs							

CAREGIVER NAME							
DATE							
🕒	MON	TUES	WED	THRS	FRI	SAT	SUN
START							
FINISH							
TOTAL Hrs							

CAREGIVER NAME							
DATE							
🕒	MON	TUES	WED	THRS	FRI	SAT	SUN
START							
FINISH							
TOTAL Hrs							

CAREGIVER NAME							
DATE							
🕒	MON	TUES	WED	THRS	FRI	SAT	SUN
START							
FINISH							
TOTAL Hrs							

_____
_____
_____

CAREGIVER TIMETABLE

CAREGIVER NAME							
DATE							
🕐	MON	TUES	WED	THRS	FRI	SAT	SUN
START							
FINISH							
TOTAL Hrs							

CAREGIVER NAME							
DATE							
🕐	MON	TUES	WED	THRS	FRI	SAT	SUN
START							
FINISH							
TOTAL Hrs							

CAREGIVER NAME							
DATE							
🕐	MON	TUES	WED	THRS	FRI	SAT	SUN
START							
FINISH							
TOTAL Hrs							

CAREGIVER NAME							
DATE							
🕐	MON	TUES	WED	THRS	FRI	SAT	SUN
START							
FINISH							
TOTAL Hrs							

_____

_____

_____

CAREGIVER TIMETABLE

CAREGIVER NAME							
DATE							
🕐	MON	TUES	WED	THRS	FRI	SAT	SUN
START							
FINISH							
TOTAL Hrs							

CAREGIVER NAME							
DATE							
🕐	MON	TUES	WED	THRS	FRI	SAT	SUN
START							
FINISH							
TOTAL Hrs							

CAREGIVER NAME							
DATE							
🕐	MON	TUES	WED	THRS	FRI	SAT	SUN
START							
FINISH							
TOTAL Hrs							

CAREGIVER NAME							
DATE							
🕐	MON	TUES	WED	THRS	FRI	SAT	SUN
START							
FINISH							
TOTAL Hrs							

_____

_____

_____

_____

CAREGIVER TIMETABLE

CAREGIVER NAME							
DATE							
🕐	MON	TUES	WED	THRS	FRI	SAT	SUN
START							
FINISH							
TOTAL Hrs							

CAREGIVER NAME							
DATE							
🕐	MON	TUES	WED	THRS	FRI	SAT	SUN
START							
FINISH							
TOTAL Hrs							

CAREGIVER NAME							
DATE							
🕐	MON	TUES	WED	THRS	FRI	SAT	SUN
START							
FINISH							
TOTAL Hrs							

CAREGIVER NAME							
DATE							
🕐	MON	TUES	WED	THRS	FRI	SAT	SUN
START							
FINISH							
TOTAL Hrs							

_____

_____

_____

CAREGIVER TIMETABLE

CAREGIVER NAME							
DATE							
🕒	MON	TUES	WED	THRS	FRI	SAT	SUN
START							
FINISH							
TOTAL Hrs							

CAREGIVER NAME							
DATE							
🕒	MON	TUES	WED	THRS	FRI	SAT	SUN
START							
FINISH							
TOTAL Hrs							

CAREGIVER NAME							
DATE							
🕒	MON	TUES	WED	THRS	FRI	SAT	SUN
START							
FINISH							
TOTAL Hrs							

CAREGIVER NAME							
DATE							
🕒	MON	TUES	WED	THRS	FRI	SAT	SUN
START							
FINISH							
TOTAL Hrs							

_____

_____

_____

CAREGIVER TIMETABLE

CAREGIVER NAME							
DATE							
🕐	MON	TUES	WED	THRS	FRI	SAT	SUN
START							
FINISH							
TOTAL Hrs							

CAREGIVER NAME							
DATE							
🕐	MON	TUES	WED	THRS	FRI	SAT	SUN
START							
FINISH							
TOTAL Hrs							

CAREGIVER NAME							
DATE							
🕐	MON	TUES	WED	THRS	FRI	SAT	SUN
START							
FINISH							
TOTAL Hrs							

CAREGIVER NAME							
DATE							
🕐	MON	TUES	WED	THRS	FRI	SAT	SUN
START							
FINISH							
TOTAL Hrs							

_____

_____

_____

SELF CARE ABILITIES

PERSONAL CARE	YES	NO	NEED ASSISTANCE	NOTES
Brush Teeth				
Change Clothes				
Bathing				
Eating				
Grooming				
Shoes On/Off				
Mobility				
Toileting				

HOME CARE	YES	NO	NEED ASSISTANCE	NOTES
Meal Prep				
Laundry				
Shopping				
Cleaning				
Transport				

SUPPORT REQUIRED

	YES	NO	NEED ASSISTANCE	NOTES

	YES	NO	NEED ASSISTANCE	NOTES

DAILY CARE LOG

NAME OF CARER		DATE	
TIME STARTED		TIME ENDED	

DUTIES CONDUCTED

MEDICATION	DOSE	TIME	NOTES	

MEALS		TIME	QUANTITY
Breakfast			
Lunch			
Snack			
Dinner			
Snack			

TIME	ACTIVITIES

PERSONAL HYGIENE	TIME	NOTES

SUPPLIES NEEDED	PURCHASED	DETAILS
○		
○		
○		

NOTES

DAILY CARE LOG

NAME OF CARER		DATE	
TIME STARTED		TIME ENDED	
DUTIES CONDUCTED			

MEDICATION	DOSE	TIME	NOTES

MEALS		TIME	QUANTITY
Breakfast			
Lunch			
Snack			
Dinner			
Snack			

TIME	ACTIVITIES

PERSONAL HYGIENE	TIME	NOTES

SUPPLIES NEEDED	PURCHASED	DETAILS
○		
○		
○		

NOTES

DAILY CARE LOG

NAME OF CARER		DATE	
TIME STARTED		TIME ENDED	

DUTIES CONDUCTED

MEDICATION	DOSE	TIME	NOTES

MEALS		TIME	QUANTITY
Breakfast			
Lunch			
Snack			
Dinner			
Snack			

TIME	ACTIVITIES

PERSONAL HYGIENE	TIME	NOTES

SUPPLIES NEEDED	PURCHASED	DETAILS
○		
○		
○		

NOTES

DAILY CARE LOG

NAME OF CARER		DATE	
TIME STARTED		TIME ENDED	
DUTIES CONDUCTED			

MEDICATION	DOSE	TIME	NOTES

MEALS		TIME	QUANTITY
Breakfast			
Lunch			
Snack			
Dinner			
Snack			

TIME	ACTIVITIES

PERSONAL HYGIENE	TIME	NOTES

SUPPLIES NEEDED	PURCHASED	DETAILS
○		
○		
○		

NOTES

DAILY CARE LOG

NAME OF CARER		DATE	
TIME STARTED		TIME ENDED	

DUTIES CONDUCTED

MEDICATION	DOSE	TIME	NOTES

MEALS		TIME	QUANTITY
Breakfast			
Lunch			
Snack			
Dinner			
Snack			

TIME	ACTIVITIES

PERSONAL HYGIENE	TIME	NOTES

SUPPLIES NEEDED	PURCHASED	DETAILS
○		
○		
○		

NOTES

DAILY CARE LOG

NAME OF CARER		DATE	
TIME STARTED		TIME ENDED	

DUTIES CONDUCTED

MEDICATION	DOSE	TIME	NOTES

MEALS		TIME	QUANTITY
Breakfast			
Lunch			
Snack			
Dinner			
Snack			

TIME	ACTIVITIES

PERSONAL HYGIENE	TIME	NOTES

SUPPLIES NEEDED	PURCHASED	DETAILS
○		
○		
○		

NOTES

DAILY CARE LOG

NAME OF CARER		DATE	
🕐 TIME STARTED		TIME ENDED	
DUTIES CONDUCTED			

MEDICATION	DOSE	TIME	NOTES

MEALS		TIME	QUANTITY
Breakfast			
Lunch			
Snack			
Dinner			
Snack			

TIME	ACTIVITIES

PERSONAL HYGIENE	TIME	NOTES

SUPPLIES NEEDED	PURCHASED	DETAILS
○		
○		
○		

NOTES

DAILY CARE LOG

NAME OF CARER		DATE	
TIME STARTED		TIME ENDED	

DUTIES CONDUCTED

MEDICATION	DOSE	TIME	NOTES

MEALS		TIME	QUANTITY
Breakfast			
Lunch			
Snack			
Dinner			
Snack			

TIME	ACTIVITIES

PERSONAL HYGIENE	TIME	NOTES

SUPPLIES NEEDED	PURCHASED	DETAILS
○		
○		
○		

NOTES

DAILY CARE LOG

NAME OF CARER		DATE	
TIME STARTED		TIME ENDED	

DUTIES CONDUCTED

MEDICATION	DOSE	TIME	NOTES	

MEALS		TIME	QUANTITY
Breakfast			
Lunch			
Snack			
Dinner			
Snack			

TIME	ACTIVITIES

PERSONAL HYGIENE	TIME	NOTES

SUPPLIES NEEDED	PURCHASED	DETAILS
○		
○		
○		

NOTES

DAILY CARE LOG

NAME OF CARER		DATE	
TIME STARTED		TIME ENDED	
DUTIES CONDUCTED			

MEDICATION	DOSE	TIME	NOTES

MEALS		TIME	QUANTITY
Breakfast			
Lunch			
Snack			
Dinner			
Snack			

TIME	ACTIVITIES

PERSONAL HYGIENE	TIME	NOTES

SUPPLIES NEEDED	PURCHASED	DETAILS
○		
○		
○		

NOTES

DAILY CARE LOG

NAME OF CARER		DATE	
TIME STARTED		TIME ENDED	

DUTIES CONDUCTED

MEDICATION	DOSE	TIME	NOTES

MEALS		TIME	QUANTITY
Breakfast			
Lunch			
Snack			
Dinner			
Snack			

TIME	ACTIVITIES

PERSONAL HYGIENE	TIME	NOTES

SUPPLIES NEEDED	PURCHASED	DETAILS
○		
○		
○		

NOTES

DAILY CARE LOG

NAME OF CARER		DATE	
TIME STARTED		TIME ENDED	

DUTIES CONDUCTED

MEDICATION	DOSE	TIME	NOTES

MEALS		TIME	QUANTITY
Breakfast			
Lunch			
Snack			
Dinner			
Snack			

TIME	ACTIVITIES

PERSONAL HYGIENE	TIME	NOTES

SUPPLIES NEEDED	PURCHASED	DETAILS
○		
○		
○		

NOTES

DAILY CARE LOG

NAME OF CARER		DATE	
TIME STARTED		TIME ENDED	
DUTIES CONDUCTED			

MEDICATION	DOSE	TIME	NOTES

MEALS		TIME	QUANTITY
Breakfast			
Lunch			
Snack			
Dinner			
Snack			

TIME	ACTIVITIES

PERSONAL HYGIENE	TIME	NOTES

SUPPLIES NEEDED	PURCHASED	DETAILS
○		
○		
○		

NOTES

DAILY CARE LOG

NAME OF CARER		DATE	
TIME STARTED		TIME ENDED	

DUTIES CONDUCTED

MEDICATION	DOSE	TIME	NOTES

MEALS		TIME	QUANTITY
Breakfast			
Lunch			
Snack			
Dinner			
Snack			

TIME	ACTIVITIES

PERSONAL HYGIENE	TIME	NOTES

SUPPLIES NEEDED	PURCHASED	DETAILS
○		
○		
○		

NOTES

DAILY CARE LOG

NAME OF CARER		DATE	
TIME STARTED		TIME ENDED	

DUTIES CONDUCTED

MEDICATION	DOSE	TIME	NOTES

MEALS		TIME	QUANTITY
Breakfast			
Lunch			
Snack			
Dinner			
Snack			

TIME	ACTIVITIES

PERSONAL HYGIENE	TIME	NOTES

SUPPLIES NEEDED	PURCHASED	DETAILS
○		
○		
○		

NOTES

DAILY CARE LOG

NAME OF CARER		DATE	
TIME STARTED		TIME ENDED	

DUTIES CONDUCTED

MEDICATION	DOSE	TIME	NOTES

MEALS		TIME	QUANTITY
Breakfast			
Lunch			
Snack			
Dinner			
Snack			

TIME	ACTIVITIES

PERSONAL HYGIENE	TIME	NOTES

SUPPLIES NEEDED	PURCHASED	DETAILS
○		
○		
○		

NOTES

DAILY CARE LOG

NAME OF CARER		DATE	
TIME STARTED		TIME ENDED	

DUTIES CONDUCTED

MEDICATION	DOSE	TIME	NOTES

MEALS		TIME	QUANTITY
Breakfast			
Lunch			
Snack			
Dinner			
Snack			

TIME	ACTIVITIES

PERSONAL HYGIENE	TIME	NOTES

SUPPLIES NEEDED	PURCHASED	DETAILS
○		
○		
○		

NOTES

DAILY CARE LOG

NAME OF CARER		DATE	
TIME STARTED		TIME ENDED	
DUTIES CONDUCTED			

MEDICATION	DOSE	TIME	NOTES

MEALS			TIME	QUANTITY
Breakfast				
Lunch				
Snack				
Dinner				
Snack				

TIME	ACTIVITIES

PERSONAL HYGIENE	TIME	NOTES

SUPPLIES NEEDED	PURCHASED	DETAILS
○		
○		
○		

NOTES

DAILY CARE LOG

NAME OF CARER		DATE	
TIME STARTED		TIME ENDED	
DUTIES CONDUCTED			

MEDICATION	DOSE	TIME	NOTES

MEALS		TIME	QUANTITY
Breakfast			
Lunch			
Snack			
Dinner			
Snack			

TIME	ACTIVITIES

PERSONAL HYGIENE	TIME	NOTES

SUPPLIES NEEDED	PURCHASED	DETAILS
○		
○		
○		

NOTES

DAILY CARE LOG

NAME OF CARER		DATE	
TIME STARTED		TIME ENDED	

DUTIES CONDUCTED

MEDICATION	DOSE	TIME	NOTES

MEALS		TIME	QUANTITY
Breakfast			
Lunch			
Snack			
Dinner			
Snack			

TIME	ACTIVITIES

PERSONAL HYGIENE	TIME	NOTES

SUPPLIES NEEDED	PURCHASED	DETAILS
○		
○		
○		

NOTES

DAILY CARE LOG

NAME OF CARER		DATE	
TIME STARTED		TIME ENDED	
DUTIES CONDUCTED			

MEDICATION	DOSE	TIME	NOTES

MEALS		TIME	QUANTITY
Breakfast			
Lunch			
Snack			
Dinner			
Snack			

TIME	ACTIVITIES

PERSONAL HYGIENE	TIME	NOTES

SUPPLIES NEEDED	PURCHASED	DETAILS
○		
○		
○		

NOTES

DAILY CARE LOG

NAME OF CARER			DATE	
TIME STARTED			TIME ENDED	

DUTIES CONDUCTED

MEDICATION	DOSE	TIME	NOTES

MEALS		TIME	QUANTITY
Breakfast			
Lunch			
Snack			
Dinner			
Snack			

TIME	ACTIVITIES

PERSONAL HYGIENE	TIME	NOTES

SUPPLIES NEEDED	PURCHASED	DETAILS
○		
○		
○		

NOTES

DAILY CARE LOG

NAME OF CARER		DATE	
TIME STARTED		TIME ENDED	

DUTIES CONDUCTED

MEDICATION	DOSE	TIME	NOTES

MEALS		TIME	QUANTITY
Breakfast			
Lunch			
Snack			
Dinner			
Snack			

TIME	ACTIVITIES

PERSONAL HYGIENE	TIME	NOTES

SUPPLIES NEEDED	PURCHASED	DETAILS
○		
○		
○		

NOTES

DAILY CARE LOG

NAME OF CARER		DATE	
TIME STARTED		TIME ENDED	

DUTIES CONDUCTED

MEDICATION	DOSE	TIME	NOTES

MEALS		TIME	QUANTITY
Breakfast			
Lunch			
Snack			
Dinner			
Snack			

TIME	ACTIVITIES

PERSONAL HYGIENE	TIME	NOTES

SUPPLIES NEEDED	PURCHASED	DETAILS
○		
○		
○		

NOTES

DAILY CARE LOG

NAME OF CARER		DATE	
TIME STARTED		TIME ENDED	

DUTIES CONDUCTED

MEDICATION	DOSE	TIME	NOTES

MEALS		TIME	QUANTITY
Breakfast			
Lunch			
Snack			
Dinner			
Snack			

TIME	ACTIVITIES

PERSONAL HYGIENE	TIME	NOTES

SUPPLIES NEEDED	PURCHASED	DETAILS
○		
○		
○		

NOTES

DAILY CARE LOG

NAME OF CARER		DATE	
TIME STARTED		TIME ENDED	

DUTIES CONDUCTED

MEDICATION	DOSE	TIME	NOTES	

MEALS		TIME	QUANTITY
Breakfast			
Lunch			
Snack			
Dinner			
Snack			

TIME	ACTIVITIES

PERSONAL HYGIENE	TIME	NOTES

SUPPLIES NEEDED	PURCHASED	DETAILS
○		
○		
○		

NOTES

DAILY CARE LOG

NAME OF CARER		DATE	
TIME STARTED		TIME ENDED	

DUTIES CONDUCTED

MEDICATION	DOSE	TIME	NOTES

MEALS		TIME	QUANTITY
Breakfast			
Lunch			
Snack			
Dinner			
Snack			

TIME	ACTIVITIES

PERSONAL HYGIENE	TIME	NOTES

SUPPLIES NEEDED	PURCHASED	DETAILS
○		
○		
○		

NOTES

DAILY CARE LOG

NAME OF CARER		DATE	
TIME STARTED		TIME ENDED	

DUTIES CONDUCTED

MEDICATION	DOSE	TIME	NOTES

MEALS		TIME	QUANTITY
Breakfast			
Lunch			
Snack			
Dinner			
Snack			

TIME	ACTIVITIES

PERSONAL HYGIENE	TIME	NOTES

SUPPLIES NEEDED	PURCHASED	DETAILS
○		
○		
○		

NOTES

DAILY CARE LOG

NAME OF CARER		DATE	
TIME STARTED		TIME ENDED	

DUTIES CONDUCTED

MEDICATION	DOSE	TIME	NOTES

MEALS		TIME	QUANTITY
Breakfast			
Lunch			
Snack			
Dinner			
Snack			

TIME	ACTIVITIES

PERSONAL HYGIENE	TIME	NOTES

SUPPLIES NEEDED	PURCHASED	DETAILS
○		
○		
○		

NOTES

DAILY CARE LOG

NAME OF CARER		DATE	
TIME STARTED		TIME ENDED	

DUTIES CONDUCTED

MEDICATION	DOSE	TIME	NOTES

MEALS		TIME	QUANTITY
Breakfast			
Lunch			
Snack			
Dinner			
Snack			

TIME	ACTIVITIES

PERSONAL HYGIENE	TIME	NOTES

SUPPLIES NEEDED	PURCHASED	DETAILS
○		
○		
○		

NOTES

DAILY CARE LOG

NAME OF CARER		DATE	
TIME STARTED		TIME ENDED	
DUTIES CONDUCTED			

MEDICATION	DOSE	TIME	NOTES

MEALS		TIME	QUANTITY
Breakfast			
Lunch			
Snack			
Dinner			
Snack			

TIME	ACTIVITIES

PERSONAL HYGIENE	TIME	NOTES

SUPPLIES NEEDED	PURCHASED	DETAILS
○		
○		
○		

NOTES

DAILY CARE LOG

NAME OF CARER		DATE	
TIME STARTED		TIME ENDED	

DUTIES CONDUCTED

MEDICATION	DOSE	TIME	NOTES

MEALS		TIME	QUANTITY
Breakfast			
Lunch			
Snack			
Dinner			
Snack			

TIME	ACTIVITIES

PERSONAL HYGIENE	TIME	NOTES

SUPPLIES NEEDED	PURCHASED	DETAILS
○		
○		
○		

NOTES

DAILY CARE LOG

NAME OF CARER		DATE	
TIME STARTED		TIME ENDED	
DUTIES CONDUCTED			

MEDICATION	DOSE	TIME	NOTES

MEALS		TIME	QUANTITY
Breakfast			
Lunch			
Snack			
Dinner			
Snack			

TIME	ACTIVITIES

PERSONAL HYGIENE	TIME	NOTES

SUPPLIES NEEDED	PURCHASED	DETAILS
○		
○		
○		

NOTES

DAILY CARE LOG

NAME OF CARER		DATE	
TIME STARTED		TIME ENDED	

DUTIES CONDUCTED

MEDICATION	DOSE	TIME	NOTES

MEALS		TIME	QUANTITY
Breakfast			
Lunch			
Snack			
Dinner			
Snack			

TIME	ACTIVITIES

PERSONAL HYGIENE	TIME	NOTES

SUPPLIES NEEDED	PURCHASED	DETAILS
○		
○		
○		

NOTES

DAILY CARE LOG

NAME OF CARER		DATE	
TIME STARTED		TIME ENDED	

DUTIES CONDUCTED

MEDICATION	DOSE	TIME	NOTES

MEALS		TIME	QUANTITY
Breakfast			
Lunch			
Snack			
Dinner			
Snack			

TIME	ACTIVITIES

PERSONAL HYGIENE	TIME	NOTES

SUPPLIES NEEDED	PURCHASED	DETAILS
○		
○		
○		

NOTES

DAILY CARE LOG

NAME OF CARER				DATE	
TIME STARTED				TIME ENDED	
DUTIES CONDUCTED					

MEDICATION	DOSE	TIME	NOTES

MEALS		TIME	QUANTITY
Breakfast			
Lunch			
Snack			
Dinner			
Snack			

TIME	ACTIVITIES

PERSONAL HYGIENE	TIME	NOTES

SUPPLIES NEEDED	PURCHASED	DETAILS
○		
○		
○		

NOTES

DAILY CARE LOG

NAME OF CARER		DATE	
TIME STARTED		TIME ENDED	
DUTIES CONDUCTED			

MEDICATION	DOSE	TIME	NOTES

MEALS		TIME	QUANTITY
Breakfast			
Lunch			
Snack			
Dinner			
Snack			

TIME	ACTIVITIES

PERSONAL HYGIENE	TIME	NOTES

SUPPLIES NEEDED	PURCHASED	DETAILS
○		
○		
○		

NOTES

DAILY CARE LOG

NAME OF CARER		DATE	
TIME STARTED		TIME ENDED	

DUTIES CONDUCTED

MEDICATION	DOSE	TIME	NOTES

MEALS		TIME	QUANTITY
Breakfast			
Lunch			
Snack			
Dinner			
Snack			

TIME	ACTIVITIES

PERSONAL HYGIENE	TIME	NOTES

SUPPLIES NEEDED	PURCHASED	DETAILS
○		
○		
○		

NOTES

DAILY CARE LOG

NAME OF CARER		DATE	
TIME STARTED		TIME ENDED	
DUTIES CONDUCTED			

MEDICATION	DOSE	TIME	NOTES

MEALS		TIME	QUANTITY
Breakfast			
Lunch			
Snack			
Dinner			
Snack			

TIME	ACTIVITIES

PERSONAL HYGIENE	TIME	NOTES

SUPPLIES NEEDED	PURCHASED	DETAILS
○		
○		
○		

NOTES

DAILY CARE LOG

NAME OF CARER		DATE	
TIME STARTED		TIME ENDED	

DUTIES CONDUCTED

MEDICATION	DOSE	TIME	NOTES

MEALS		TIME	QUANTITY
Breakfast			
Lunch			
Snack			
Dinner			
Snack			

TIME	ACTIVITIES

PERSONAL HYGIENE	TIME	NOTES

SUPPLIES NEEDED	PURCHASED	DETAILS
○		
○		
○		

NOTES

DAILY CARE LOG

NAME OF CARER		DATE	
TIME STARTED		TIME ENDED	
DUTIES CONDUCTED			

MEDICATION	DOSE	TIME	NOTES

MEALS		TIME	QUANTITY
Breakfast			
Lunch			
Snack			
Dinner			
Snack			

TIME	ACTIVITIES

PERSONAL HYGIENE	TIME	NOTES

SUPPLIES NEEDED	PURCHASED	DETAILS
○		
○		
○		

NOTES

DAILY CARE LOG

NAME OF CARER		DATE	
TIME STARTED		TIME ENDED	

DUTIES CONDUCTED

MEDICATION	DOSE	TIME	NOTES

MEALS		TIME	QUANTITY
Breakfast			
Lunch			
Snack			
Dinner			
Snack			

TIME	ACTIVITIES

PERSONAL HYGIENE	TIME	NOTES

SUPPLIES NEEDED	PURCHASED	DETAILS
○		
○		
○		

NOTES

DAILY CARE LOG

NAME OF CARER		DATE	
TIME STARTED		TIME ENDED	

DUTIES CONDUCTED

MEDICATION	DOSE	TIME	NOTES

MEALS		TIME	QUANTITY
Breakfast			
Lunch			
Snack			
Dinner			
Snack			

TIME	ACTIVITIES

PERSONAL HYGIENE	TIME	NOTES

SUPPLIES NEEDED	PURCHASED	DETAILS
○		
○		
○		

NOTES

DAILY CARE LOG

NAME OF CARER		DATE	
TIME STARTED		TIME ENDED	
DUTIES CONDUCTED			

MEDICATION	DOSE	TIME	NOTES

MEALS		TIME	QUANTITY
Breakfast			
Lunch			
Snack			
Dinner			
Snack			

TIME	ACTIVITIES

PERSONAL HYGIENE	TIME	NOTES

SUPPLIES NEEDED	PURCHASED	DETAILS
○		
○		
○		

NOTES

DAILY CARE LOG

NAME OF CARER		DATE	
TIME STARTED		TIME ENDED	

DUTIES CONDUCTED

MEDICATION	DOSE	TIME	NOTES

MEALS		TIME	QUANTITY
Breakfast			
Lunch			
Snack			
Dinner			
Snack			

TIME	ACTIVITIES

PERSONAL HYGIENE	TIME	NOTES

SUPPLIES NEEDED	PURCHASED	DETAILS
○		
○		
○		

NOTES

DAILY CARE LOG

NAME OF CARER		DATE	
TIME STARTED		TIME ENDED	

DUTIES CONDUCTED

MEDICATION	DOSE	TIME	NOTES

MEALS		TIME	QUANTITY
Breakfast			
Lunch			
Snack			
Dinner			
Snack			

TIME	ACTIVITIES

PERSONAL HYGIENE	TIME	NOTES

SUPPLIES NEEDED	PURCHASED	DETAILS
○		
○		
○		

NOTES

DAILY CARE LOG

NAME OF CARER		DATE	
TIME STARTED		TIME ENDED	
DUTIES CONDUCTED			

MEDICATION	DOSE	TIME	NOTES

MEALS		TIME	QUANTITY
Breakfast			
Lunch			
Snack			
Dinner			
Snack			

TIME	ACTIVITIES

PERSONAL HYGIENE	TIME	NOTES

SUPPLIES NEEDED	PURCHASED	DETAILS
○		
○		
○		

NOTES

DAILY CARE LOG

NAME OF CARER		DATE	
TIME STARTED		TIME ENDED	

DUTIES CONDUCTED

MEDICATION	DOSE	TIME	NOTES

MEALS		TIME	QUANTITY
Breakfast			
Lunch			
Snack			
Dinner			
Snack			

TIME	ACTIVITIES

PERSONAL HYGIENE	TIME	NOTES

SUPPLIES NEEDED	PURCHASED	DETAILS
○		
○		
○		

NOTES

DAILY CARE LOG

NAME OF CARER		DATE	
TIME STARTED		TIME ENDED	

DUTIES CONDUCTED

MEDICATION	DOSE	TIME	NOTES

MEALS		TIME	QUANTITY
Breakfast			
Lunch			
Snack			
Dinner			
Snack			

TIME	ACTIVITIES

PERSONAL HYGIENE	TIME	NOTES

SUPPLIES NEEDED	PURCHASED	DETAILS
○		
○		
○		

NOTES

DAILY CARE LOG

NAME OF CARER		DATE	
TIME STARTED		TIME ENDED	

DUTIES CONDUCTED

MEDICATION	DOSE	TIME	NOTES

MEALS		TIME	QUANTITY
Breakfast			
Lunch			
Snack			
Dinner			
Snack			

TIME	ACTIVITIES

PERSONAL HYGIENE	TIME	NOTES

SUPPLIES NEEDED	PURCHASED	DETAILS
○		
○		
○		

NOTES

DAILY CARE LOG

NAME OF CARER		DATE	
TIME STARTED		TIME ENDED	

DUTIES CONDUCTED

MEDICATION	DOSE	TIME	NOTES

MEALS		TIME	QUANTITY
Breakfast			
Lunch			
Snack			
Dinner			
Snack			

TIME	ACTIVITIES

PERSONAL HYGIENE	TIME	NOTES

SUPPLIES NEEDED	PURCHASED	DETAILS
○		
○		
○		

NOTES

DAILY CARE LOG

NAME OF CARER		DATE	
TIME STARTED		TIME ENDED	

DUTIES CONDUCTED

MEDICATION	DOSE	TIME	NOTES

MEALS		TIME	QUANTITY
Breakfast			
Lunch			
Snack			
Dinner			
Snack			

TIME	ACTIVITIES

PERSONAL HYGIENE	TIME	NOTES

SUPPLIES NEEDED	PURCHASED	DETAILS
○		
○		
○		

NOTES

DAILY CARE LOG

NAME OF CARER		DATE	
TIME STARTED		TIME ENDED	
DUTIES CONDUCTED			

MEDICATION	DOSE	TIME	NOTES

MEALS		TIME	QUANTITY
Breakfast			
Lunch			
Snack			
Dinner			
Snack			

TIME	ACTIVITIES

PERSONAL HYGIENE	TIME	NOTES

SUPPLIES NEEDED	PURCHASED	DETAILS
○		
○		
○		

NOTES

DAILY CARE LOG

NAME OF CARER		DATE	
TIME STARTED		TIME ENDED	

DUTIES CONDUCTED

MEDICATION	DOSE	TIME	NOTES

MEALS		TIME	QUANTITY
Breakfast			
Lunch			
Snack			
Dinner			
Snack			

TIME	ACTIVITIES

PERSONAL HYGIENE	TIME	NOTES

SUPPLIES NEEDED	PURCHASED	DETAILS
○		
○		
○		

NOTES

DAILY CARE LOG

NAME OF CARER		DATE	
TIME STARTED		TIME ENDED	
DUTIES CONDUCTED			

MEDICATION	DOSE	TIME	NOTES

MEALS		TIME	QUANTITY
Breakfast			
Lunch			
Snack			
Dinner			
Snack			

TIME	ACTIVITIES

PERSONAL HYGIENE	TIME	NOTES

SUPPLIES NEEDED	PURCHASED	DETAILS
○		
○		
○		

NOTES

DAILY CARE LOG

NAME OF CARER		DATE	
TIME STARTED		TIME ENDED	

DUTIES CONDUCTED

MEDICATION	DOSE	TIME	NOTES

MEALS		TIME	QUANTITY
Breakfast			
Lunch			
Snack			
Dinner			
Snack			

TIME	ACTIVITIES

PERSONAL HYGIENE	TIME	NOTES

SUPPLIES NEEDED	PURCHASED	DETAILS
○		
○		
○		

NOTES

DAILY CARE LOG

NAME OF CARER		DATE	
TIME STARTED		TIME ENDED	

DUTIES CONDUCTED

MEDICATION	DOSE	TIME	NOTES	

MEALS			TIME	QUANTITY
Breakfast				
Lunch				
Snack				
Dinner				
Snack				

TIME	ACTIVITIES

PERSONAL HYGIENE	TIME	NOTES	

SUPPLIES NEEDED	PURCHASED	DETAILS	
○			
○			
○			

NOTES

DAILY CARE LOG

NAME OF CARER		DATE	
TIME STARTED		TIME ENDED	
DUTIES CONDUCTED			

MEDICATION	DOSE	TIME	NOTES

MEALS		TIME	QUANTITY
Breakfast			
Lunch			
Snack			
Dinner			
Snack			

TIME	ACTIVITIES

PERSONAL HYGIENE	TIME	NOTES

SUPPLIES NEEDED	PURCHASED	DETAILS
○		
○		
○		

NOTES

DAILY CARE LOG

NAME OF CARER		DATE	
TIME STARTED		TIME ENDED	

DUTIES CONDUCTED

MEDICATION	DOSE	TIME	NOTES

MEALS			TIME	QUANTITY
Breakfast				
Lunch				
Snack				
Dinner				
Snack				

TIME	ACTIVITIES

PERSONAL HYGIENE	TIME	NOTES

SUPPLIES NEEDED	PURCHASED	DETAILS
○		
○		
○		

NOTES

DAILY CARE LOG

NAME OF CARER		DATE	
TIME STARTED		TIME ENDED	

DUTIES CONDUCTED

MEDICATION	DOSE	TIME	NOTES

MEALS		TIME	QUANTITY
Breakfast			
Lunch			
Snack			
Dinner			
Snack			

TIME	ACTIVITIES

PERSONAL HYGIENE	TIME	NOTES

SUPPLIES NEEDED	PURCHASED	DETAILS
○		
○		
○		

NOTES

DAILY CARE LOG

NAME OF CARER		DATE	
TIME STARTED		TIME ENDED	

DUTIES CONDUCTED

MEDICATION	DOSE	TIME	NOTES

MEALS		TIME	QUANTITY
Breakfast			
Lunch			
Snack			
Dinner			
Snack			

TIME	ACTIVITIES

PERSONAL HYGIENE	TIME	NOTES

SUPPLIES NEEDED	PURCHASED	DETAILS
○		
○		
○		

NOTES

DAILY CARE LOG

NAME OF CARER		DATE	
TIME STARTED		TIME ENDED	

DUTIES CONDUCTED

MEDICATION	DOSE	TIME	NOTES

MEALS		TIME	QUANTITY
Breakfast			
Lunch			
Snack			
Dinner			
Snack			

TIME	ACTIVITIES

PERSONAL HYGIENE	TIME	NOTES

SUPPLIES NEEDED	PURCHASED	DETAILS
○		
○		
○		

NOTES

DAILY CARE LOG

NAME OF CARER		DATE	
TIME STARTED		TIME ENDED	

DUTIES CONDUCTED

MEDICATION	DOSE	TIME	NOTES

MEALS		TIME	QUANTITY
Breakfast			
Lunch			
Snack			
Dinner			
Snack			

TIME	ACTIVITIES

PERSONAL HYGIENE	TIME	NOTES

SUPPLIES NEEDED	PURCHASED	DETAILS
○		
○		
○		

NOTES

DAILY CARE LOG

NAME OF CARER		DATE	
TIME STARTED		TIME ENDED	
DUTIES CONDUCTED			

MEDICATION	DOSE	TIME	NOTES

MEALS		TIME	QUANTITY
Breakfast			
Lunch			
Snack			
Dinner			
Snack			

TIME	ACTIVITIES

PERSONAL HYGIENE	TIME	NOTES

SUPPLIES NEEDED	PURCHASED	DETAILS
○		
○		
○		

NOTES

DAILY CARE LOG

NAME OF CARER		DATE	
TIME STARTED		TIME ENDED	

DUTIES CONDUCTED

MEDICATION	DOSE	TIME	NOTES

MEALS		TIME	QUANTITY
Breakfast			
Lunch			
Snack			
Dinner			
Snack			

TIME	ACTIVITIES

PERSONAL HYGIENE	TIME	NOTES

SUPPLIES NEEDED	PURCHASED	DETAILS
○		
○		
○		

NOTES

DAILY CARE LOG

NAME OF CARER		DATE	
TIME STARTED		TIME ENDED	|ует
DUTIES CONDUCTED			

MEDICATION	DOSE	TIME	NOTES

MEALS		TIME	QUANTITY
Breakfast			
Lunch			
Snack			
Dinner			
Snack			

TIME	ACTIVITIES

PERSONAL HYGIENE	TIME	NOTES

SUPPLIES NEEDED	PURCHASED	DETAILS
○		
○		
○		

NOTES

DAILY CARE LOG

NAME OF CARER		DATE	
TIME STARTED		TIME ENDED	

DUTIES CONDUCTED

MEDICATION	DOSE	TIME	NOTES

MEALS		TIME	QUANTITY
Breakfast			
Lunch			
Snack			
Dinner			
Snack			

TIME	ACTIVITIES

PERSONAL HYGIENE	TIME	NOTES

SUPPLIES NEEDED	PURCHASED	DETAILS
○		
○		
○		

NOTES

DAILY CARE LOG

NAME OF CARER		DATE	
TIME STARTED		TIME ENDED	
DUTIES CONDUCTED			

MEDICATION	DOSE	TIME	NOTES

MEALS		TIME	QUANTITY
Breakfast			
Lunch			
Snack			
Dinner			
Snack			

TIME	ACTIVITIES

PERSONAL HYGIENE	TIME	NOTES

SUPPLIES NEEDED	PURCHASED	DETAILS
○		
○		
○		

NOTES

DAILY CARE LOG

NAME OF CARER		DATE	
TIME STARTED		TIME ENDED	

DUTIES CONDUCTED

MEDICATION	DOSE	TIME	NOTES

MEALS		TIME	QUANTITY
Breakfast			
Lunch			
Snack			
Dinner			
Snack			

TIME	ACTIVITIES

PERSONAL HYGIENE	TIME	NOTES

SUPPLIES NEEDED	PURCHASED	DETAILS
○		
○		
○		

NOTES

DAILY CARE LOG

NAME OF CARER		DATE	
TIME STARTED		TIME ENDED	

DUTIES CONDUCTED

MEDICATION	DOSE	TIME	NOTES

MEALS		TIME	QUANTITY
Breakfast			
Lunch			
Snack			
Dinner			
Snack			

TIME	ACTIVITIES

PERSONAL HYGIENE	TIME	NOTES

SUPPLIES NEEDED	PURCHASED	DETAILS
○		
○		
○		

NOTES

DAILY CARE LOG

NAME OF CARER		DATE	
TIME STARTED		TIME ENDED	

DUTIES CONDUCTED

MEDICATION	DOSE	TIME	NOTES

MEALS		TIME	QUANTITY
Breakfast			
Lunch			
Snack			
Dinner			
Snack			

TIME	ACTIVITIES

PERSONAL HYGIENE	TIME	NOTES

SUPPLIES NEEDED	PURCHASED	DETAILS
○		
○		
○		

NOTES

DAILY CARE LOG

NAME OF CARER			DATE	
TIME STARTED			TIME ENDED	

DUTIES CONDUCTED

MEDICATION	DOSE	TIME	NOTES

MEALS		TIME	QUANTITY
Breakfast			
Lunch			
Snack			
Dinner			
Snack			

TIME	ACTIVITIES

PERSONAL HYGIENE	TIME	NOTES

SUPPLIES NEEDED	PURCHASED	DETAILS
○		
○		
○		

NOTES

DAILY CARE LOG

NAME OF CARER		DATE	
TIME STARTED		TIME ENDED	
DUTIES CONDUCTED			

MEDICATION	DOSE	TIME	NOTES

MEALS		TIME	QUANTITY
Breakfast			
Lunch			
Snack			
Dinner			
Snack			

TIME	ACTIVITIES

PERSONAL HYGIENE	TIME	NOTES

SUPPLIES NEEDED	PURCHASED	DETAILS
○		
○		
○		

NOTES

DAILY CARE LOG

NAME OF CARER		DATE	
TIME STARTED		TIME ENDED	|ожно

DUTIES CONDUCTED

MEDICATION	DOSE	TIME	NOTES

MEALS		TIME	QUANTITY
Breakfast			
Lunch			
Snack			
Dinner			
Snack			

TIME	ACTIVITIES

PERSONAL HYGIENE	TIME	NOTES

SUPPLIES NEEDED	PURCHASED	DETAILS
○		
○		
○		

NOTES

DAILY CARE LOG

NAME OF CARER		DATE	
TIME STARTED		TIME ENDED	

DUTIES CONDUCTED

MEDICATION	DOSE	TIME	NOTES

MEALS		TIME	QUANTITY
Breakfast			
Lunch			
Snack			
Dinner			
Snack			

TIME	ACTIVITIES

PERSONAL HYGIENE	TIME	NOTES

SUPPLIES NEEDED	PURCHASED	DETAILS
○		
○		
○		

NOTES

DAILY CARE LOG

NAME OF CARER		DATE	
TIME STARTED		TIME ENDED	

DUTIES CONDUCTED

MEDICATION	DOSE	TIME	NOTES	

MEALS		TIME	QUANTITY
Breakfast			
Lunch			
Snack			
Dinner			
Snack			

TIME	ACTIVITIES

PERSONAL HYGIENE	TIME	NOTES

SUPPLIES NEEDED	PURCHASED	DETAILS
○		
○		
○		

NOTES

DAILY CARE LOG

NAME OF CARER		DATE	
TIME STARTED		TIME ENDED	

DUTIES CONDUCTED

MEDICATION	DOSE	TIME	NOTES

MEALS		TIME	QUANTITY
Breakfast			
Lunch			
Snack			
Dinner			
Snack			

TIME	ACTIVITIES

PERSONAL HYGIENE	TIME	NOTES

SUPPLIES NEEDED	PURCHASED	DETAILS
○		
○		
○		

NOTES

DAILY CARE LOG

NAME OF CARER		DATE	
TIME STARTED		TIME ENDED	

DUTIES CONDUCTED

MEDICATION	DOSE	TIME	NOTES

MEALS		TIME	QUANTITY
Breakfast			
Lunch			
Snack			
Dinner			
Snack			

TIME	ACTIVITIES

PERSONAL HYGIENE	TIME	NOTES

SUPPLIES NEEDED	PURCHASED	DETAILS
○		
○		
○		

NOTES

DAILY CARE LOG

NAME OF CARER		DATE	
TIME STARTED		TIME ENDED	

DUTIES CONDUCTED

MEDICATION	DOSE	TIME	NOTES

MEALS		TIME	QUANTITY
Breakfast			
Lunch			
Snack			
Dinner			
Snack			

TIME	ACTIVITIES

PERSONAL HYGIENE	TIME	NOTES

SUPPLIES NEEDED	PURCHASED	DETAILS
○		
○		
○		

NOTES

DAILY CARE LOG

NAME OF CARER		DATE	
TIME STARTED		TIME ENDED	

DUTIES CONDUCTED

MEDICATION	DOSE	TIME	NOTES

MEALS		TIME	QUANTITY
Breakfast			
Lunch			
Snack			
Dinner			
Snack			

TIME	ACTIVITIES

PERSONAL HYGIENE	TIME	NOTES

SUPPLIES NEEDED	PURCHASED	DETAILS
○		
○		
○		

NOTES

DAILY CARE LOG

NAME OF CARER		DATE	
TIME STARTED		TIME ENDED	
DUTIES CONDUCTED			

MEDICATION	DOSE	TIME	NOTES

MEALS		TIME	QUANTITY
Breakfast			
Lunch			
Snack			
Dinner			
Snack			

TIME	ACTIVITIES

PERSONAL HYGIENE	TIME	NOTES

SUPPLIES NEEDED	PURCHASED	DETAILS
○		
○		
○		

NOTES

DAILY CARE LOG

NAME OF CARER		DATE	
TIME STARTED		TIME ENDED	

DUTIES CONDUCTED

MEDICATION	DOSE	TIME	NOTES

MEALS		TIME	QUANTITY
Breakfast			
Lunch			
Snack			
Dinner			
Snack			

TIME	ACTIVITIES

PERSONAL HYGIENE	TIME	NOTES

SUPPLIES NEEDED	PURCHASED	DETAILS
○		
○		
○		

NOTES

DAILY CARE LOG

NAME OF CARER		DATE	
TIME STARTED		TIME ENDED	
DUTIES CONDUCTED			

MEDICATION	DOSE	TIME	NOTES

MEALS		TIME	QUANTITY
Breakfast			
Lunch			
Snack			
Dinner			
Snack			

TIME	ACTIVITIES

PERSONAL HYGIENE	TIME	NOTES

SUPPLIES NEEDED	PURCHASED	DETAILS
○		
○		
○		

NOTES

DAILY CARE LOG

NAME OF CARER		DATE	
TIME STARTED		TIME ENDED	

DUTIES CONDUCTED

MEDICATION	DOSE	TIME	NOTES

MEALS		TIME	QUANTITY
Breakfast			
Lunch			
Snack			
Dinner			
Snack			

TIME	ACTIVITIES

PERSONAL HYGIENE	TIME	NOTES

SUPPLIES NEEDED	PURCHASED	DETAILS
○		
○		
○		

NOTES

NOTES

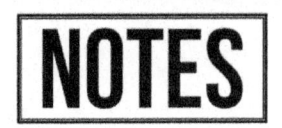

NOTES

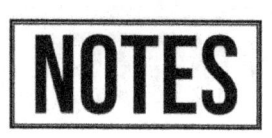

NOTES

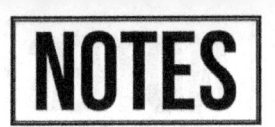

NOTES

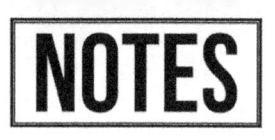

Made in the USA
Columbia, SC
04 January 2024